THYROID THERAPY GUIDE

Treatment For Balancing Hormones And Energy Levels

Fine-Tune Your Thyroid Function With Therapies That Balance Hormones And Boost Overall Energy Levels

DR. BRIDGET PROMISE

Table of Contents

CHAPTER ONE

Introduction

Thyroid Tune-Up is an all-encompassing resource that provides insight into the optimization of thyroid health. Throughout this expedition, we shall examine the critical significance of energy levels and hormonal equilibrium, delving into the complex anatomical and physiological aspects of the thyroid gland.

By producing hormones, the thyroid is essential for the maintenance of numerous physiological functions; any disruption in this process can result in common conditions such as hypothyroidism. To attain a more comprehensive comprehension of the thyroid and its influence on general health, we shall commence this investigation.

The Significance Of Energy Levels And Hormonal Balance

Hormones function as intra-organic mediators, controlling a multitude of physiological processes to preserve equilibrium and harmony. Out of the hormones in question, those generated by the thyroid gland exert the most substantial impact on metabolism, energy generation, and general vitality.

Thyroid hormones, more precisely thyroxine (T4) and triiodothyronine (T3) play a critical role in regulating the metabolic rate of the body. The process through which the body transforms sustenance into energy, known as metabolism, is vital for life. Optimal thyroid function regulates this energy production to maintain a delicate equilibrium, preventing either an excess or deficiency.

Ensuring hormonal equilibrium is critical for maintaining consistent energy levels over the day. When thyroid function is optimal, individuals can maintain a consistent energy level, which empowers them to engage in routine activities with renewed strength and eagerness. Conversely, disruptions in energy levels can result from imbalances in thyroid hormones; these symptoms include fatigue, lethargy, and a general feeling of malaise.

Comprehension Of Thyroid Operation

The thyroid gland, situated in the anterior region of the neck, is a diminutive organ in the form of a butterfly that regulates energy expenditure and metabolism. Hormones produced by this endocrine gland have an extensive impact on all cells, tissues, and organs within the body.

Physiology And Anatomy Of The Thyroid Gland

To fully grasp the intricacies of the thyroid, an investigation into its anatomy and physiology is imperative. Two lobes of thyroid tissue are joined by a narrow band of tissue known as the isthmus. Situated near the trachea and just below the larynx, also known as the voice box, the thyroid is ideally positioned to monitor and react to fluctuations in the metabolic demands of the body.

The ability of the thyroid gland to absorb iodine from the circulation and use it to produce thyroid hormones is unparalleled. Iodine is an essential constituent in the biosynthesis of the two principal hormones secreted by the thyroid, thyroxine (T4) and triiodothyronine (T3).

After being released into the circulation, these hormones proceed to regulate metabolism in a variety of tissues and organs.

CHAPTER TWO

Function Of Thyroid Hormones Within The Human Body

Thyroid hormones manifest their physiological effects through a variety of mechanisms. Among their principal functions is the regulation of the metabolic rate, which governs the rate at which energy is generated from nutrients within the body.

An optimally operating thyroid is responsible for maintaining a steady metabolic rate, which facilitates the effective utilization of energy obtained from food.

In particular, thyroid hormones are essential for the development and maturation of organs and tissues during infancy and adolescence. They exert an influence on cardiovascular system functionality, thereby affecting both pulse rate and blood pressure.

Furthermore, thyroid hormones play a crucial role in the regulation of body temperature, guaranteeing that it stays within the ideal range necessary for the proper functioning of physiological processes.

Frequent Thyroid Conditions

Despite its complex architecture and intrinsic regulatory mechanisms, the thyroid is vulnerable to a range of disorders that have the potential to impair its functionality. Hypothyroidism, an extremely common thyroid disorder, is distinguished by the presence of an underactive thyroid gland.

The Causes, Symptoms, And Diagnosis Of Hypothyroidism

When the thyroid gland fails to produce adequate quantities of thyroid hormones to meet the demands of the body, hypothyroidism ensues. The development of hypothyroidism may be influenced by various factors, such as autoimmune diseases, genetic susceptibility, and specific medications.

Hypothyroidism is characterized by fatigue, weight gain, temperature sensitivity, thin skin, and hair loss, among other symptoms. Due to their pivotal function in metabolism regulation, insufficiency of thyroid hormones may cause a deceleration in metabolic processes, thereby manifesting the aforementioned distinctive symptoms.

A comprehensive assessment of symptoms, physical examination, and laboratory tests are required to diagnose hypothyroidism. To assess thyroid function, blood assays quantify concentrations of thyroid-stimulating hormone (TSH), unbound thyroxine (T4), and triiodothyronine (T3). In many cases, increased TSH levels are indicative of a hypoactive thyroid, which necessitates additional testing and diagnosis.

We have undertaken an exploration of the complexities surrounding thyroid health in Thyroid Tune-Up, with a particular focus on the importance of hormonal equilibrium and energy levels in the preservation of general wellness.

A comprehensive comprehension of the intricacies of thyroid hormones and the anatomy and physiology of the thyroid gland will enable individuals to acquire an understanding of the delicate equilibrium necessary for achieving optimal health.

Our investigation has also encompassed hypothyroidism, a prevalent thyroid disorder that impacts a substantial number of people globally. An understanding of the etiology, manifestations, and diagnostic approaches associated with hypothyroidism is vital for individuals aiming to effectively treat and control this condition.

Keep in mind that as we further explore the realm of thyroid health, knowledge is a potent instrument for proactive wellness. The purpose of Thyroid Tune-Up is to provide readers with the necessary information to effectively navigate the intricate aspects of thyroid health and initiate a path towards optimal health and equilibrium.

Identifying Indications Of Hyperthyroidism And Pursuing Treatment

A condition distinguished by an excessively active thyroid gland, hyperthyroidism is brought about by an overproduction of the thyroid hormones thyroxine (T4) and triiodothyronine (T3).

A small butterfly-shaped organ situated in the neck, the thyroid gland regulates energy production, metabolism, and numerous other physiological processes. An overactive thyroid is associated with a variety of symptoms that impact numerous body systems.

CHAPTER THREE

Identification Of Indicators Of Hyperthyroidism

The timely detection of hyperthyroidism is critical to implement effective treatment and intervention. Though the manifestations of hyperthyroidism can differ, the following are frequent indicators:

1. Unexplained weight loss can occur in individuals with hyperthyroidism, despite the presence of a normal or increased appetite.

2. Elevated Heart Rate: Symptoms of an overactive thyroid include a

heightened heart rate, palpitations, and occasionally irregular heart rhythms; these manifestations may exacerbate symptoms of anxiety and restlessness.

3. Heat Intolerance and Excessive Sweating: Individuals with hyperthyroidism may develop an intolerance to heat and excessive sweating, causing them to feel uncomfortably heated in ambient temperatures.

4. Fatigue and muscular Weakness: Individuals diagnosed with hyperthyroidism frequently express feelings of fatigue and

muscular weakness, despite their elevated energy expenditure.

5. Diarrhoea and alterations in gastrointestinal habits are symptoms of hyperthyroidism that can have an impact on the digestive system.

6. Irritability and mood swings are both influenced by thyroid hormones, which also impact emotional health. An overabundance of these hormones may result in agitation, irritability, anxiety, or panic attacks.

7. Disruptions to Sleep: People diagnosed with hyperthyroidism may experience challenges

initiating or maintaining sleep, which can result in insomnia and general fatigue.

Tools For Diagnosis And Tests:

Healthcare personnel employ a variety of diagnostic instruments and tests to validate a diagnosis of hyperthyroidism and ascertain its fundamental etiology. Possible examples include:

1. Comprehensive Overview of Thyroid Function Tests

The utilization of thyroid function assays is essential for determining the blood concentrations of thyroid hormones. The principal assays comprise the quantification of thyroid stimulating hormone (TSH), T3, and T4. In conjunction with low TSH, elevated levels of T3 and T4 are indicative of hyperthyroidism. These tests serve as a foundational measure for assessing the extent of the ailment and informing decisions regarding treatment.

2. Imaging Methods for the Assessment of the Thyroid

The evaluation of the thyroid gland's structure and function is significantly aided by imaging. Thyroid scintigraphy and radioactive iodine uptake (RAIU) are two nuclear medicine examinations that can be utilized to detect nodules or regions of heightened activity within the thyroid. These scans assist in ascertaining the etiology of hyperthyroidism, including potential underlying factors such as Graves' disease or thyroid nodules.

3. Methods that Consider the Thyroid Wholely

Although traditional medical procedures are frequently required, incorporating holistic methodologies can enhance medical treatments and promote thyroid health as a whole.

Nutrition And Dietary Support For The Thyroid

The thyroid functions in dependence on specific nutrients; therefore, maintaining thyroid health through a balanced diet is possible. Beneficial foods include those that are abundant in iodine, selenium, zinc, and omega-3 fatty acids. A registered dietitian or healthcare professional should be consulted, however, to ensure that dietary modifications are to one's specific health requirements.

Lifestyle and Physical Activity to Improve Thyroid Function:

It is well known that consistent physical activity improves thyroid function. Physical activity can aid in weight management, metabolic enhancement, and the alleviation of hyperthyroidism symptoms. Nevertheless, maintaining a healthy equilibrium is critical, as overexertion may worsen specific symptoms and should be evaluated by a medical professional.

CHAPTER FOUR

Traditional Therapies

1. Antithyroid Pharmaceuticals:

Methimazole and propylthiouracil are examples of antithyroid drugs that function by impeding the synthesis of thyroid hormones.

Frequently prescribed, these drugs restore thyroid hormone levels to normal and alleviate symptoms. Consistent thyroid function monitoring is imperative when it comes to medication management.

2. Radiation-induced iodine therapy:

Radioactive iodine therapy consists of the oral administration of radioactive iodine, which destroys overactive thyroid cells through selective targeting. While frequently employed to treat Graves' disease, this approach carries the risk of inducing hypothyroidism, which necessitates everlasting replacement of thyroid hormone.

3. Performing a thyroidectomy:

When alternative therapies prove ineffective or in severe cases, surgical excision of the thyroid gland, in its entirety or part, may be advised. A definitive treatment option, thyroidectomy necessitates everlasting replacement therapy with thyroid hormone.

In conclusion, it is imperative to promptly seek medical attention upon identifying the symptoms of hyperthyroidism to ensure effective management. Healthcare professionals utilize diagnostic tools, such as imaging techniques and thyroid function tests, to ascertain the underlying cause and extent of the condition. In conjunction with conventional treatments, holistic methodologies, including exercise and appropriate nutrition, can contribute to a more holistic and well-rounded approach to thyroid health. Traditional therapies, such as thyroidectomy, radioactive iodine therapy, and antithyroid medications, are designed to restore thyroid function to normal levels and mitigate associated symptoms. Achieving successful management of hyperthyroidism and promoting overall well-being ultimately requires a collaborative approach between healthcare providers and patients.

A considerable proportion of the worldwide populace is afflicted with thyroid disorders, which frequently necessitate a combination of surgical procedures, pharmaceutical interventions, and alternative treatment modalities for optimal management.

During this discourse, we shall examine the diverse methodologies employed to tackle thyroid disorders, encompassing traditional pharmaceuticals, surgical interventions, and non-pharmaceutical approaches such as acupuncture, botanical remedies, and stress management strategies.

Therapeutic Agents For Thyroid Disorders

Medication-induced regulation of hormone levels constitutes a fundamental approach to treating thyroid complications. Thyroid hormones are primarily composed of thyroxine (T4) and triiodothyronine (T3). To supplement deficient hormone levels, patients with hypothyroidism, a condition characterized by an underactive thyroid, frequently receive synthetic thyroid hormones like levothyroxine. By aiding in the restoration of thyroid hormone homeostasis, this medication alleviates symptoms including cold sensitivity, fatigue, and weight gain.

Conversely, pharmaceutical interventions that impede the synthesis of thyroid hormones may be prescribed to patients with hyperthyroidism, a condition characterized by an overactive thyroid. Methimazole and propylthiouracil are anti-thyroid medications that function by inhibiting the thyroid gland's capacity to generate excessive quantities of hormones. The primary objectives of these medications are to restore thyroid hormone levels to a healthy state and alleviate symptoms such as anxiety, weight loss, and tachycardia.

Surgical Procedures And Interventions

When pharmaceutical interventions are inadequate or complications arise, surgical interventions might be taken into consideration. Thyroidectomy, the surgical elimination of a portion or the entirety of the thyroid gland, is a frequent operation.

Individuals with thyroid cancer, large goiters, or severe

hyperthyroidism that does not respond well to medication may be advised to undergo this treatment.

Although thyroid surgery is frequently a highly effective treatment, it frequently necessitates the long-term administration of thyroid hormone replacement medications. Risks associated with surgery also include potential injury to adjacent structures, including the vocal cords and parathyroid glands.

Contrary Therapies

To supplement the management of thyroid disorders, numerous

individuals investigate alternative therapies in addition to conventional treatments. These alternative methodologies prioritize comprehensive wellness and frequently incorporate acupuncture, herbal remedies, and mind-body integration.

CHAPTER FIVE

Herbal Supplements For Thyroid Health

For thyroid support, herbs and natural supplements are frequently considered. Asha, bladderwrack, and guggul are common botanicals that are thought to have beneficial effects on thyroid function.

As an adaptogenic herb, ashwagandha is believed to assist in hormone homeostasis and tension relief, both of which can negatively affect thyroid health. Iodine, which is present in bladderwrack, a variety of seaweed, is an essential constituent in the synthesis of thyroid hormone. Research has examined the potential of guggul, which is obtained from the resin of the mukul myrrh tree, to provide support for thyroid function.

Before integrating herbal remedies into a treatment regimen, it is imperative to exercise prudence and seek guidance from healthcare professionals, given the potential for drug interactions and individual contraindications.

Acupuncture And The Medicine Of Traditional China

Acupuncture, which has its origins in Traditional Chinese Medicine (TCM), is an increasingly recognized alternative therapy utilized for the treatment of thyroid disorders. The body is regarded as an interconnected network of energy pathways according to Traditional Chinese Medicine, and the goal of acupuncture is to restore Qi balance to the body. Acupuncture may assist in regulating thyroid function and alleviating symptoms associated with thyroid disorders, according to some studies.

Although acupuncture exhibits potential, further investigation is required to definitively ascertain its efficacy. Akin to herbal remedies, individuals contemplating acupuncture ought to seek guidance from their healthcare providers to ascertain whether it harmonizes with their comprehensive treatment regimen.

Mind-Body Relationship

The interrelation between the mind and body is vital for overall health, which includes thyroid function. The endocrine system can be influenced by stress, anxiety, and emotional well-being, which in turn can affect the secretion of thyroid hormone. The potential of mind-body practices, including yoga, meditation, and deep-breathing exercises, to mitigate stress and promote thyroid health is becoming increasingly acknowledged.

Techniques For Stress Management To Promote Thyroid Harmony

Thyroid disorders may be exacerbated or developed in part as a result of chronic stress. Techniques for stress management seek to lessen the physiological effects of tension to foster a state of equilibrium and tranquility. Engaging in mindfulness and meditation can assist individuals in developing a state of tranquility, which may have advantageous effects on thyroid function.

Yoga, which emphasizes breathing regulation, physical postures, and meditation, is an additional effective method of stress management. Consistent engagement in yoga has been linked to enhancements in a multitude of physical and mental health parameters, including the alleviation of tension.

By stimulating the body's relaxation response, deep breathing exercises (pranayama or diaphragmatic breathing) can counteract the effects of the stress hormone cortisol. The incorporation of these practices into one's daily routine may potentially promote thyroid health by fostering a more harmonious relationship between the mind and body.

In summary, the treatment of thyroid disorders involves an extensive array of strategies, including traditional pharmaceuticals, surgical procedures, and alternative healing modalities. Acupuncture, herbal remedies, and stress management techniques provide patients with supplementary alternatives to consider in conjunction with their medical practitioners.

For optimal thyroid health outcomes, patients must collaborate closely with medical professionals to develop a comprehensive treatment plan that is individualized to their specific requirements and conditions.

CHAPTER SIX

Mental Health And Its Influence On Thyroid Function

The correlation between the mind and body is indisputable, and psychological well-being has a substantial impact on the intricate regulation of hormones (including those generated by the thyroid) in the body.

Endocrine system disruptions caused by chronic stress, anxiety, and depression may impact the synthesis and control of thyroid hormones.

Particularly, stress induces the secretion of cortisol, a hormone linked to the fight-or-flight response in the body. Prolonged increases in cortisol levels have the potential to impede the transformation of dormant thyroid hormone (T4) into its active form (T3), thereby resulting in diminished thyroid functionality. Moreover, inflammation induced by stress may have adverse effects on the thyroid gland, thereby further impairing its capacity to operate at its peak.

Hence, comprehending and effectively handling tension constitute an essential component in preserving thyroid well-being. The daily integration of stress-relieving activities into one's routine, including yoga, meditation, and deep-breathing exercises, has the potential to enhance thyroid function and mental health.

Thyroid-Friendly Meal Plans And Recipes

The function of diet in promoting thyroid health is crucial. A thyroid-friendly diet must consist primarily of nutrient-dense meals that supply vital vitamins and minerals. Sample meal plans and nutrient-dense recipes intended to support thyroid function are provided in this article, which also promotes hormonal balance.

Recipes Packed With Nutrients To Promote Thyroid Health

1. Salmon and Seaweed Salad: This salad promotes thyroid function and cardiovascular health in general due to its high iodine and omega-3 fatty acid content.

2. Quinoa Spinach Bowl: Brimming with B vitamins, magnesium, and iron, this bowl aids in the fight against fatigue which is frequently the result of thyroid imbalances.

3. Roasted Brazil Nut Mix: Selenium, an essential mineral for thyroid health, is abundant in Brazil nuts. Together with other nuts and seeds, they produce a savory and nutritious nibble when roasted.

Meal Plans Illustrative Of Balanced Hormones

Day 1:

• Greek yogurt parfait with berries and walnuts for breakfast.

• Grilled chicken salad accompanied by avocado and quinoa for lunch

Baked salmon served with asparagus and sweet potatoes for supper

Day 2:

• Spinach and feta omelet with whole grain toast for breakfast

• Lentil and Vegetable Soup Served with Mixed Greens as a Side Dish

• Tofu stir-fried with broccoli and brown rice for supper

The provided sample meal plans prioritize a diverse selection of nutrient-dense foods, thereby guaranteeing a balanced and comprehensive diet that promotes optimal thyroid function.

Nutritional Supplements And Nutraceuticals

Although a nutritious diet serves as the fundamental basis for thyroid health, specific nutraceuticals, and supplements may offer supplementary assistance. Comprehension of vital nutrients that support the thyroid, as well as judicious selection and application of supplements, are integral elements of a holistic approach to thyroid care.

CHAPTER SEVEN

Vital Nutrients To Support The Thyroid

1. Iodine, which is essential for the synthesis of thyroid hormone, is present in dairy products, fish, and algae.

2. Selenium, an exceptionally potent antioxidant, facilitates the transformation of T4 to T3. Turkey, Brazil almonds, and sunflower seeds are all outstanding sources.

3. Vitamin D, which is indispensable for thyroid health and immune function, can be

acquired via supplementation or solar exposure.

4. Zinc, which is essential for the production of thyroid hormone, is found in foods such as pumpkin seeds, beef, and shellfish.

Caution In Selecting And Employing Supplements

Before integrating dietary supplements into one's routine, it is imperative to seek guidance from a healthcare professional to ascertain specific requirements and identify any possible drug interactions. Optimal dietary supplements procured from reputable manufacturers guarantee that the body exclusively absorbs the desired advantages, devoid of superfluous additives or contaminants.

Individual Narratives Of Thyroid Recovery

True-life experiences that aim to restore vitality and hormonal equilibrium offer motivation and inspiration to individuals who are grappling with their thyroid health obstacles.

Thyroid Warrior Testimonials Of Inspiration

1. In "Sabecca's Story: Overcoming Hypothyroidism Through Diet and

Lifestyle Changes," the author Sarah recounts her journey of revitalizing her health and vitality via stress management and mindful eating.

2. In "John's Journey: Thriving with Hyperthyroidism by Embracing a Holistic Approach," the author John recounts the profound impact that the adoption of a holistic lifestyle—encompassing judicious nutrition and diligent self-care—had on his hyperthyroidism experience.

Conclusion

This investigation's overriding objective is to enable readers to assume authority over their thyroid health. By acquiring knowledge regarding the influence of mental health on thyroid function, adopting thyroid-friendly recipes, integrating nutrient-dense foods into their daily diets, and exercising discernment when selecting supplements, individuals may initiate a process that results in hormonal equilibrium and long-lasting vitality.

Concluding Remarks and Best Wishes for a Dynamic and Spacious Life

To conclude this discourse, we encourage readers to adopt a conscientious and conscientious approach toward their thyroid health, recognizing that even minor adjustments to their way of life can yield substantial enhancements. May this information inspire and guide you toward living a life filled with vitality and vigor?

www.ingramcontent.com/pod-product-compliance
Lightning Source LLC
Chambersburg PA
CBHW071107260726
48661CB00006B/2513